I0414886

From
Conversations
With
The
Boys
revised

Johnnie Newkirk, Jr.

ISBN: 0-7596-0253-0 (e)

ISBN: 0-7596-0254-9 (sc)

Printed in the United States of America
Bloomington, IN

This book is printed on acid free paper.

1st Books - rev. 4/4/2006

Johnnie Newkirk Jr.
In
Association
With
New West Music & Publishing Inc.
WWW.NEWWESTMUSICPUBLISHING.COM
PO BOX 250670
Brooklyn, N.Y. 11225
718-469-6432

Catalogue nwpb002

DEDICATED

TO

THE

BOYS

COMMENT

These are *only* some of the Opinions, Thoughts and Creative Ideas that have been shared by me, and with me, and others, over the years. These are <u>not</u> facts, and should <u>not</u> be seen, or taken, as such.

Author

WARNING

Due to the <u>mature/adult</u> nature of <u>some</u> of the material in this book, it is <u>not</u> suitable, nor is it suggested reading, for anyone under 18 years of age. As with everything else in life, <u>always</u> exercise common-sense; <u>always</u> practice safe-sex; <u>always</u> follow the law; and <u>don't</u> do, or engage in anything, or <u>any</u> activity, that could result in <u>any</u> physical, emotional, or legal harm/ anguish to you, or to anyone else. This can be done by <u>always</u> respecting yourself, others, the law, and your environment.

Author

While she's in the kitchen stirring the stew, and you're both walking around in your Birthday Suits- embrace her from behind- and use your "Love Tool" to plug up any hole of which she gives her consent.

Position yourself behind her, remove her Bra, and with the use of your hands- cup her Breasts- and with the use of your fingers, work on her Nipples until the lady decides to "Confess."

While looking at her *Clitoris*, sing to it that tune that Barry White made so famous: "You're my first, my last, my everything."

When making love, while the music is playing in the background, always *"hump* and *pump"* to the beat of the Bass.

Make having Sex with *you* her "Addiction."

Never play your trump-card with your woman.

Become familiar with her natural "body-odor."

Does she like to engage in "rough sex?" And- if she does, how rough? Remember: When she says enough- stop!

Foreplay is an "Art," so master it.

When she tells you, "why you cannot be more like John," arrange for her to be *with* John.

As often as your wallet will permit, redecorate your bedroom. This will make you feel like you're making "love" in a *new* place.

Never, ever embarrass your woman in public.

From time to time, give your "love-making" a theme.

Never smack, or hit, your woman unless it's with *your* "love-tool."

When you finger-pop a woman, always use a condom. This will greatly cut the risk of any infection.

Love and respect your woman, but never *more* than you love and respect yourself.

Periodically, take a vacation from engaging in any type of sexual activity.

Tickle her, tickle her you know where. If you don't know where, she'll guide you there. If you *do* tickle her in said place, she'll spring open her 'gap," and you'll have an *"ejaculating"* day. Now you know why *no* bedroom should be without a Feather!

There are quite a few women who prefer their meat *tart*, not sweet.

Create your own *Sexual Trademark.*

Create your own *Sexual Slogan.*

Always make your woman feel *safe* and *secure.*

Never let a woman get into your bed, *unless* she intends to spread her legs.

Always reassure her that *your* body is *hers*, and it's always available for her pleasure.

Find out what part of *your* anatomy your woman is *most* attracted to.

Guys remember: It's dangerous to mess with *another* man's pleasure.

Let your woman know that her *natural* body smell, helps to keep *you* under *her* "Spell."

Fulfill a *sexual* desire of hers' that *very* few others would be willing, or able, to fulfill.

For all you guys that are *quite* well endowed, and have a problem finding a condom that fits- buy yourselves a box of *Latex Sanitary Gloves.* Hey! I hear it does the trick.

It is "sexually beneficial" for all concerned, if you would change *your* "sexual-style" from time to time.

You should, from time to time, put on a "strip- tease" show for your woman, and make each show even more *creative,* and *exciting,* than the last one.

Let her perform *oral-sex* on you, while you're standing on your head. Yes!

I find that a woman's nose can be quite "erotic."

Call her on the phone, and tell her in a soft, firm, but masculine voice, what you intend to do too her, and with her, sexually, when you get home.

If you're a breast man, bring home *breasts*; If you're a leg man, bring home *legs*; But, do not bring home something you dislike, and be constantly critical of it.

The truth will often *kill* the *thrill.*

Never lie to her, just don't *always* give her an answer.

Peroxide: There should not be a bedroom without it.

If you're a man, and have a little girl in you, do not let your woman see it.

If your woman ever ask you, if you've ever had sex with another man- look at her, as if she's crazy, and continue to watch T.V.

If you record your sexual encounters, *erase* them as soon as possible.

When she's performing oral-sex on you, inform her to apply a lot of *suction*- especially, just before you're about to ejaculate.

Even if it has been "mutually agreed" beforehand, don't penetrate her while she is sleeping. It is better to be safe, than sorry. Because, people, *too* often, forget that which was previously agreed.

Always make sure that she's provided for.

Dirty talk is the *best* Aphrodisiac.

Never neglect one part of *her* anatomy for another.

If you *must* cheat, please see that *safe-sex* is practiced by *all* parties involved.

Drugs, and Alcohol, and Sex just does not mix.

Never discuss your woman, sexually, with *anyone*. I mean this literally.

Ask her how *she* likes to be kissed.

Healthy teeth, gums, and clean breath are a *must*.

There isn't anything wrong with being "*sexually selfish*" from time to time.

If you want to know what women are thinking, read *some* of what they read.

Your *tongue* holds a lot of bacteria, so *never* forget to brush your tongue along with your teeth.

Don't forget to floss your teeth on a daily basis.

Take special care of your lips, for they are quite sensuous.

Have you ever performed the *"sixty-nine"* position, in the standing position?

Take some fruit syrup, and apply some to her earlobes. While you're sucking on them with your lips, rim her inner ears with your tongue, and watch the sparks fly.

Guys: Unless you're willing to participate in a "three-some" with another man, don't insist on a "three-some" with another woman. This, basically, pertains to heterosexual couples.

What do women, and, a lot of homosexuals have in common? They are *both*, usually, on the receiving end.

How come women can refer to their female friends as their "girlfriends" and men cannot refer to their male friends as their "boyfriends?" Whatever happened to "what is good for the Goose, is also good for the Gander?"

When a Woman says "N0," don't you go there. Don't go there *today*; Don't go there *tomorrow*; And, if you were smart, you didn't go there *yesterday*.

"The truth hurts." This is what a friend would always say to someone when he felt that they were being less than truthful, with him, about themselves. What he fails to realize, however, is that the "truth" is often- times personal, and <u>should</u> be kept private. For society will usually take <u>your</u> truth, and use it against you at a later date.*r*

Hey, guys: If what's good for the Goose, is also good for the Gander, then women must, also, understand that the same rules must apply too them when we say "NO." But, when do we ever say No?

Guys: There isn't anything wrong with making your woman squirm from time to time. They have been doing that to us for years.

How about writing a *RAP* song for your woman, and, if it's not X-Rated, maybe you could have a hit song on your hand.

The best way for you and your woman to understand each other, is to *"role-play."*

While still inside of her, without slipping out of her, make a complete 180° turn. Oh! How sweet it is.

Pick a certain night of the week when you will treat *your* woman, as if she is nothing more than *your* personal "whore."

Before you start to engage in sexual intercourse-sit down with your mate, and have a serious discussion about *birth-control, and abortion.*

If you remember nothing else, *please* remember this: *hiv, and Aids, are "no" joke.*

There are a lot of *Sexually Transmitted Diseases* out there, which are too numerous to mention here. So, go to the library with your mate, get a book on the subject, and familiarize yourselves with the different types of STD's out there. Learn. Don't get burned.

Let's become great lovers *first*, and get that out of the way, then we can concentrate on becoming the best of friends.

Learn to *Love* each other; *Lust* after one another; and *Laugh* with each other.

I do not condone the practice of "golden-showers." However, if that's your thing: drink plenty of water, shower together before, and after, and avoid any open wounds.

Couples should go to bed for only *two* reasons: and watching television shouldn't be one of them.

Hey guys, women love men with *round, firm* and *robust* rear-ends. So, do what you have to do to develop a "butt" that *really* matters.

Once you've penetrated her, and you're inside of her, stay in there while you're sleeping – even if it's "all night long."

If you must be an "octopus," at least touch all the right spots.

Invent your own sexual positions, and give them each an original name.

There's a time to be gentle, and there's a time to be rough. But, when in doubt, follow her lead.

Don't you dare to compare, if *you* wish to keep on docking there.

If she wants to wear your clothes- let her. If you want to wear hers- don't!

If you want to impress your woman, then pay attention to all the *small* details.

Hey guys, make a choice: Do you want to sleep with your mate, *or* your "Ego?"

Don't lock yourself in by *your* own definitions: By talking a good Talk, and *not* walking a good Walk.

When you're making Love you want to be left alone; so please do not forget to disconnect the telephone.

If you like using soap, please use one that has a *mild* spring scent to it.

Remember: Her *breasts* are special, so *each* one should have their own name.

No pets allowed. They may be *your* best friend, but they may not, necessarily, be hers.

If your woman tends to analyze your relationship to death, remind her that you're *not* in a psychology- class, and that, that type of behavior is a "turn-off."

Why not play a game of "horse-shoes," and let her toss some horse-shoes on to, *your, "erect"* *horse.*

Where a woman is concerned, and sex is involved, *never* "presume," or "assume" anything. Ask!

Invest in *flannel sheets* for the winter, and *satin sheets* for the summer.

If you want to keep "slicing" that behind, you better not forget her when it's Valentines'.

Always control your "love-tool," and don't *ever* let it control you.

Remember: Never discuss *business* in bed. It's bad for sex.

Concentrate more on "loving" her, and less on "pleasing" her, and you'll come out ahead on both fronts. Because to love, is too please.

Take the time, and the patience needed to learn your woman's <u>*erogenous zones.*</u>

Learn how to, and practice massaging your mate's buttocks.

Learn how to, and practice massaging your mate's stomach.

Boys, you don't need that cologne. Trust me!

Make love to her in an open, isolated field-during a summer shower.

Periodically, have a "No Clothes" weekend. This way you both can reacquaint yourselves with each other's body.

Remember guys: *Belching and blowing gas in bed is a turn-off, and not seductive at all.*

Foreplay, sexual-intercourse, and after-play: What you lack in one area, you can *make up,* for, in the others.

Sleeping with a *Friend* is like playing the "stock-market:" Risky business.

Learn and practice the Art of Licking. It's more satisfying to lick the rim, before you put it in.

Let her smell that manly musk, on *your* manly "tusk."

Never bring up her past, *especially,* in bed.

Once we get into a *steady* relationship, we tend to stop flirting with our lady. Hey, flirt with her. Try it. She'll like it.

Don't be afraid to be *"child-like"* with your woman. It's O.K. to rest your head in her Lap.

The *body* is a beautiful thing. So tell me: Why *all* the tattoos? Why *all* the piercing?

When doing it *"doggie-style,"* during the deep strokes - spank her ever so softly on her buns, to the down strokes of your drum.

Remember: Good sex doesn't always lead to *Romance*, and good romance doesn't always lead to good *Sex*.

If you're over-sexed, *please,* do not get a woman that's under-sexed.

Outside, the bedroom, appreciate her for her mind. Inside, the bedroom, appreciate her for her body.

Yes, it is true. There are quite a number of women who like to be used.

You have your *Lips*, your *Tongue*, your *Hands* and your *Love-Tool*, of which all- simultaneously at times- should be used to take care of the "business" at hand.

Forget about asking her about her astrological sign, because, it doesn't, and shouldn't, matter.

If a woman tells you: "no romance without finance," then she shouldn't be the woman for you.

A woman is beautiful *with,* or *without,* her clothes on, so, enjoy the view.

When she has to ask, *"Where's The Beef,"* this is when you should realize there's a problem.

Show me a "man" that says he *knows* women, and I'll show you a liar.

If she is *good* enough to perform "oral-sex" on you, then she is, also, *good* enough to be *kissed* by you afterwards.

Your *teeth* are very important, so visit your Dentist on a regular basis.

If you're hungry- nibble on her. If she's hungry, let her nibble on you.

Instead of taking a lunch break, why not take a "*lust*" break.

If you do not wear underwear, beware of the *zipper,* especially, if you're *not* circumcised. Ouch!

What you discuss with your "friends," *don't* discuss, with your woman.

After an early morning workout, treat yourselves to a "*champagne and strawberry*" brunch.

She can't make *you* feel "sexy," if *you* don't feel sexy already.

If she charges you for *her* "sexual favors," then charge her for *yours,* as well. After all: Let it be known that "your worth" is equivalent to "hers."

If you *must* sweat- fine. But, don't you ever *beg* for a "Piece of Leg."

Say it; Believe it; Achieve it. You are what *you* say you are. You can do what *you* say you can do.

Plant your face between her naked thighs, and *smell* the aroma; take *delight* in the aroma; and become *intoxicated* by the aroma.

Don't *sweat* it, if she doesn't want to *swallow* it.

If *you're* satisfied with the size of *your* "penis," so will she, or he. One never knows!

Homosexuality: Something that *many* want to experience; quite a *few* want to practice on a regular basis; but no one wants to admit to it- not even to themselves.

Remember: Good *foreplay* guarantees you sex, today. Good after-play guarantees you sex, another day.

The issue of *one's* sexuality is a very sensitive one. I strongly, and sincerely, believe that some people are truly confused about *who* and *what* they want sexually. This is why it's so important *not* to force them into *any* particular role by labeling them.

Let her know when you're itching, and then *show* her where to scratch.

Buy a pair of *edible* underwear, and have her eat the *whole* thing.

In this day and age, I definitely do not advocate "Group Sex," for the stakes are just *too* high.

Talk to her breasts: Who knows, they may answer you back.

Hold one of her breasts in your hand, pretend that it's a microphone, and start singing into it. How about singing the hit song "Get Ready," by the Temptations, cause, here you come.

Save your money; join a *health club*; and workout. It will do wonders for your "self-esteem," and it will do wonders for your sex-life.

If the heels on your shoes are worn down, and your shoes aren't shined- women will *usually* assume *two* things: You're probably not *too* particular about your appearance, and your pockets are probably quite empty.

Before you decide to swing from a "chandelier," make sure that said chandelier can *support* your weight.

Find an *isolated* area on a beach, and have a race- in the *nude*- with your mate. The winner gets to perform, or have you perform, whatever sexual acts that they desire.

Warning: Engaging in sex, while driving, can be *hazardous* to your health.

This is something that I do not, at all, advocate. But if you must use a woman- or a man for that matter- don't abuse them. In essence: If you *must* use, at least, *don't* abuse.

Why not practice CPR- especially mouth to mouth resuscitation. This will not only be quite Educational, but, Inspirational and Enjoyable as well.

It's summer time, and you, and your mate, are sitting on a *tree* branch, in the nude, just touching and kissing each other, while enjoying the "summer breeze."

Do your *Aerobic* exercises in the nude.

He likes to have his fingernails manicured, and painted. He likes to have his toenails pedicure and painted. He, also, get his eyebrows waxed, and he's, somewhat, effeminate. However, he isn't considered "Gay." What is he considered: Metro-sexual.

Using *sex* as a guideline, play the game: "Simon Says." This can also be a "group event."

She's facing you, sitting on your shoulders with her legs wrapped around your neck, and you're performing "oral-sex" on her. What a blast!

You'll be surprised with what you can do with a *cleaned,* unpeeled, semi-ripe green plantain.

It's unfortunate, but true: A lot of guys lack *"finesse."*

If you stay in *shape, dress well* and carry yourself in manly fashion- women *will, usually,* find you attractive, even if yours looks aren't all that.

Find out *all* of her Fetishes, and share *all* of yours with her.

Remember: Your friends, today, can be your enemies tomorrow, and the reverse holds true. So be extremely careful of whom you trust, what you trust them with, and of whom, and to whom you criticize. If it isn't something pleasant, don't say it.

Once in awhile, I'll make it quite clear to my lady, especially on the down-stroke, that there is no-one better for *Thee* than *Me*. The truth will set her free!

"Behind every great man there is a great woman." Translations: The woman can be great, as long as, she remains "behind" the man.

America: "Land of the brave and home of the free." Translation: Those who are brave are the ones who are entitled, and deserve to be, free. All "cowards" need not, and should not, apply.

If she's a "Virgin," and your feelings for her aren't sincere, *please,* do not take her "cherry."

KY-Jelly: No home should be without it.

Remember that there's a Slot out there that *will* fit *your* Machine.

Once a month, pay for her to go to the beauty salon of *her* choice. Hey! *You* won't look good, if she doesn't look good.

When she no longer returns your calls, call someone else. Don't be like that poor mouse who had only one, *clean,* hole to go into.

If you *must* run a line on her make sure *you,* and only *you*, are its' author.

Wouldn't it be thrilling to "bungee-jump" in the "raw."

There is a sexual practice that I, definitely, don't recommend: It's called "urethral intercourse." Why would anyone want to engage in, or even consider engaging in, such an act is completely, beyond, comprehension.

If you have *any* doubt that performance doesn't count, then evidently you have never heard this: He isn't S__ in bed. Hey, need I say more.

Believe it, or not: Women love *our* "rods" just as much as we love their "pods." And that's a fact.

I *like* older women because they teach me. I *love* younger women because I teach them.

A *kept* man is *not* a "Man." This is not an opinion, this is a fact.

When you go out with your lady, please leave your "homeboys" at home.

Imagine having oral sex being performed on you while you're riding on the Cyclone, and you *start* to 'ejaculate," just prior to that *deep* drop. Wow!

If she wants to learn how to drive a "Standard," then let your "love tool" be the "stick shift." Oh, I love how she "*shift,*" those gears!

While under the *clear* beach waters of the Bahamas, take turns performing oral sex on each other.

Picture this: You're outdoors with, your lady, you're both slow dancing, in the raw, under a clear, blue "summer moon." Oh what a night!

It's not a reflection on her, but I value my *space* and my *solitude.*

Women *aren't* satisfied unless they know what *you're* always thinking.

They'll deny it, but if a guy is *too* nice, a woman will, inevitably, take advantage of him.

The *less* I see of her, the *more* attractive, and desirable, she becomes.

If you do not respond to *her* advances, why must *you* be "gay," and everything else *she* calls you.

If you *won't* give "head," then there's no need for you to be in, *my,* bed.

A lot of guys are becoming more "strictly-dickly." I, on the other hand, will remain "strictly- clitley." And you can take that, "clitorally."

If you want to score, go to an *all* male strip-show. Cause the women *will* be "Hot" to go. Think about it!

No one can "read" a woman better than an *"out"* of the closet gay.

Making love in the nude, on a warm, summer night, on "tar beach (roof top)."

I do miss the "Orgies" of *yester years.*

Many women do subscribe, to men who *aren't* circumcised.

Let's be honest guys: Some of us, do, at times, like being spanked by our mates.

He may be "Gay," but what makes *you* feel that *he,* necessarily, wants *you!* Don't flatter yourself.

When I see a woman with her "Ass" on her shoulder, I go out of *my* way to sleep with her, *just* to "dog her." Someone needs to bring women like that back *down* to "earth."

It's has been *rumored* that "gays" give the best "head." I love good "head." How about you?

There is, another, growing practice that I don't particularly care for, and it's when someone derives gratification, and satisfaction, from eating the feces of their sexual partner. This should be a warning to be very careful,, and selective, about whom you "kiss."

Women sure can be *rough* with our "balls." Easy, baby. Easy!

Guys, if we're going to be true to ourselves, we know we have more "Crap" with *us*, then "women," and "gays," combined.

If, "anal-sex" is *your* game, then don't forget this, important, name: Enema. Buy it; Use it; Stock it.

You've satisfied her, *financially*; You've satisfied her, *emotionally*; You've, even, satisfied her, *sexually*. Now, after doing all that satisfying, she's still not satisfied. Why? Because you were too busy doing all the above, that you didn't spent enough, quality, time with her.

There is nothing wrong with *loving* "sex." Just choose your partners carefully, and practice *"Safe-Sex."*

Most guys aren't, weak; they're just not, *very,* strong. You show me a *really* strong man, and I'll show you a "man" that, *generally,* walks alone.

Guys: Don't let *anyone* tell you how much "sex" is *too* much for you. Remember: If you don't *use* it, you'll *lose* it.

Women hate to be called the "B" word, but they have *no* problem with calling "men" *everything*, other than their "God" given n

If you're not out there committing *crimes*, using *drugs*, abusing *alcohol,* or puffing on *cigarettes*- your "masculinity" is questioned- and you're made to feel like you're less than a "man." This is *classic* "peer- pressure."

At times, I feel that we live in an "era" where men cannot do anything *correct*- as if to say: Up with women, and down with men!

If you have to spray something on it, just to keep it *erect*, then you need to see a doctor. Word!

I wish my woman would stop worrying about being *my* "personal slut," and just *go* ahead, and, *be* it.

Making love, in the nude, on top of a *"highway billboard."* Oh what a thrill! Oh what a rush!

A man is like a *mouse*: He's not satisfied until he's been *in,* and *ou,* of every hole.

When you're *tired*, let your fingers do *your* talking, and, if she doesn't like it, then let her feet do *her* walking.

Women pretend *so* much, you wonder if you're really, *ever,* satisfying them.

Women will *always* play the role of the "Victim,' and love it.

If she is willing to be the "master- chef," in the *bedroom*, then I'm willing to be the "master-chef," in the *kitchen*.

Men want *good* sex. Women want the whole nine yards.

Believe it, or not, there are quite a few individuals who derive pleasure, and gratification, from being defecated on by their sexual partners. This is know as: "brown showers"

Convince your woman that it's alright to come to bed, once in awhile, all made up.

I *"love,"* my "home-boy," and I "love you": Two different types of *relationships*, and two, *completely,* different types of love. So, let's dispense with any jealousy.

Unlike *some* men, I don't mind my woman being a *little* "tomboyish."

In the privacy of our home, I want her to be *my* topless waitress.

Tell her: Keep your "friends' *out* of my bedroom, and I'll stay *out* of theirs.

Variety, from the same person, is *not* the type of variety I'm talking about, looking for, or want.

If you *insist* on listening to your "friends,' then I must, insist, that you go, and be with *them*.

Educate your woman about the sports *you* love.

If you are a heterosexual male, and want to engage in a sexual experience with another guy, follow these simple rules: A) Make sure the guy acts like a guy. B) Lives in another state. C) Practice and engage in safe, and protective, sex. D) Donot give out your Name, Rank, or Serial Number- simply put: don't know me, cause, I don't know you. E) Never, ever tell a sole- not even yourself. F) If all else fails, deny, deny, deny.

I find *nothing* attractive, nor sexy, about female "body- builders."

If you ever have the slightest doubt about anyone that you have had, or wish to have, an intimate, or sexual, relationship, or encounter with, do absolutely nothing! When in doubt, sit it out.

I don't want to get married; I don't want to live with anyone; and my *career* comes first. Hey, it works for me!

What's my order of preference: oral; anal; and vaginal-intercourse. What's your order of preference?

To make out all night in a deserted "cave,' is a real turn-on for me. How about you?

If I'm *all* that "negative," then why are you, still, with me?

Why do "men' feel, the *need* to measure their Penis?

Wouldn't it be wonderful to go see the skating on ice, and discover that *all* the performers are performing in, the raw. It doesn't get any "cooler" than that.

Picture this: You, and your mate, are in an empty roller dome, and you're "roller-skating" in the nude to the music of *your* choice. Wow!

When you "spot" someone observing your "erect" penis, just let them know that it's alright, and just say to them, what "Humphrey Bogart" said in Casablanca: "Here's looking at you kid." Say this while pointing your, still, "erect" penis in their direction.

Just dreaming of *different* ways to satisfy her, and myself for that matter, gives me a "euphoric" feeling.

The only *positive* thing about being physically ill is having *her* nursing me back to "good health."

Pretend I'm Santa Claus, sit in the nude on old Santa's lap, and tell old Santa what you want for Christmas. Ho! Ho! Ho!

In *general*, women just cannot be trusted.

A mistress will satisfy that part of you that you *usually* will not, or cannot, let your wife satisfy.

Don't play "dumb" just to placate me. I find that quite insulting, and quite degrading, and I *will,* eventually, resent you for it.

Do you know what's surprisingly sad: Older women play *more* mind games, than those that are much younger than they are.

Women are *always* complaining that there aren't any *good* "men" out there. Well, the feeling is mutual.

I wonder how it would feel to engage in sexual intercourse on the Patio of my apartment complex- "all night long."

My woman loves it when I take a fresh, firm strawberry, and use it to *massage* her Clitoris, and then use it to *penetrate* her vagina. Do I eat it afterwards? Yes! Remember: Waste not, want not.

I would love to build a "tree house' where me, and my lady, can go when we want our *privacy.*

Wouldn't it be a *thrill*- for you and your mate- to engage in '"sexual intercourse" while suspended in "mid-air." Remember: The sky is the limit.

There isn't anything *wrong*, or *queer*, with a woman massaging *her* "man's" buns.

When I'm in bed, I'm considered a "Great Communicator."

Unless I have a desire to sleep with the man, I don't give a damn what *his* "sexual preference" is. So, why do you care?

If you've hit *hard* times "financially," would you sleep with another man? Most guys will answer "No," and most will be lying. The truth hurts.

Since I don't believe that "leopards" change *their* spots, I could never marry an ex-prostitute. But you can if you want to.

I have *no* problem with being a "freak," just as long as it is with another *"consenting" adult.* I do not like to pass judgment- but *anyone* who would engage in *any* sexual activity with *any* "minor," or *any* "animal-" is "sick."

Today, more than yesterday, I *long* for a "virgin."

How come women love to "match-make?"

Women can be quite mean, but I've *learned*- when the need presents itself- to be just as mean, or even, more so.

With regards to "ugly women": Never insult them, and never, ever pay them a compliment; for if you do either, you'll live to regret it.

Men speak through the use of *their* bodies; Women speak through the use of *their* tongues. However, I was taught that *"talk"* is cheap, and that *"actions"* speaks louder than words. I like the way "men" speak.

To me, an intelligent woman who *retains,* and *maintains,* her "femininity," is not only quite attractive, but quite "sexy" as well.

Listen ladies: Sex is something I *want*. It's not, necessarily, something I *need*.

Let your "condoms" be your "life support:" *Don't* go anywhere without them.

Tell your woman, from time to time, what makes *her* "unique" out of bed, as well as, in bed.

Before you sleep with each other, get a complete physical, and a complete blood-work. When you *both* get your clean bill of health, *still* practice "safe-ex," but keep your *past* sexual experiences to yourself. Because, what one doesn't know, in this case, won't hurt them. For today should be the *first* day of *your* life.

It might sound *corny,* and it might sound *rude*, but if you don't do it, then you are a "fool." Say to her point blank: If you want to be with *me*, you'll have to show *me* some I.D. Remember that looks are deceiving, and the tongue tells a lot of lies.

I can think of a way in which you, and your mate, can engage in face to face, oral- sex; face to face, vaginal-intercourse, and, anal-intercourse- while you *both* are swinging on a "swing." How about you?

When I no longer consider a woman a "sex object," I no longer consider that woman desirable.

When I *know* that my woman is *definitely* trying to screw me over, I, usually, take my *hard* "love-tool," and slide it up her "ass." It's her pain, but my gain. Because, this lets her know who is in control. And she *never, ever* resist.

Do not limit yourself by just dating women of your own race, or nationality. For, in this instance, "variety" is, the "spice of life."

Let's be honest. We don't want to be "gay," but quite a few of us wouldn't mind "cracking" the behinds of some of those "softies" with our *long* and *robust* "love-tool." It's a shame, but, too many of them just talk *too* much. So, one is afraid to give them a "taste of the honey." And even if you gave them a taste, they'd get greedy, and keep coming back for more. Forget it!

You're both standing, engaging in sexual intercourse in the missionary position, and you're riding on the merry-go-round. Wow.

Introduce people to "*you,*" before you introduce them to, *your,*" sexuality."

Close your eyes, and tell me what you <u>feel,</u> and what you <u>see</u>. Also, tell me *how* you would *like* to <u>feel</u>, and *what* you would *like* to <u>see</u>. And I'll do everything, within my power, to make *both* of them come true.

We're in the *center field* of a major league stadium. We are making love in the "doggie style" position, and it's a hot, clear, summer's night. The stadium is empty, and all of the stadium lights are on. Do I know how to score, or, do I know how to score. Yes!

It has been *rumored* that "gays-" in general, give the *best* "head," and that "bisexuals-" in general, are usually the *best* "lovers" in bed. If this has, any, validity, then it makes one wonder: What are "heterosexuals" best at?

Instead of viewing "sex" between *consenting adults,* as being "diverse," too many people would rather view it as, being, "perverted."

Buy a small, battery operated massager, and use it to massage *all* of her "nooks and crannies."

Love and tolerance works hand in hand. For you cannot have one without the other.

"It's not the size of the "ship," but the motion of the ocean. This is what the *not* so well endowed tell those that are *well* endowed to placate themselves.

When the "ball" drops on New Year's Eve, so should *your* load, if you catch my drip!

Whatever you have thought about, sexually, has already been thought of, and done, by others. Translation: You're not alone.

Freak: An individual who has the *guts* to explore their "sexual fantasies," without allowing themselves to be labeled by others, as long as, said acts are between *consenting adults.*

Whatever *my* woman wants me to do, to satisfy her sexually, I will. However, if she isn't willing to do the same for me, then it will be time, for me, too set her free!

Have a wrestling match in the Mud, with your mate, and when it's over, make love in the Mud.

Engage in a "kissing marathon" with your mate.

While you're giving her a ride on the *"bar"* of your bike, have her perform oral- sex on you.

"The only thing a man can do for me, is show me where the omen are."

Never over estimate, or under estimate, *your* worth- either in, or out of, bed.

Men *must* learn to do what women have, basically, always done: embrace each other, "emotionally."

When you walk in on a *naked* woman, the first things that she covers, are her breasts, and, not her vaginal area. Why?

In one's bedroom I, also, believe there should he a *separation* of "church and state."

We are, basically, here on this planet for *two* reasons: to Learn, and to Love. I intend to *keep* on learning, and I, also, intend too *keep* on loving.

There are those that state that "homosexuality" has a *negative* effect on the "family structure." If this is so, then what effect, does the following, have on said "family structure:" A) Adultery, B) Single Parent Households, C) Divorce, and D) Teen Pregnancy? You be the judge.

Unfortunately, a lot of men subscribe to this old adage: "Where women are concerned, I believe in the *three* "Fs": Find them; F... them; and Forget them.

Beauty is not only "skin deep," it's "heart deep," as well.

Love is not blind, but, the heart usually is.

I believe that "sexual statistic" are, the most misleading statistic of all.

If the "talk shows" are any indication, we are a "love starved" society.

Some of the prettiest women that I've ever seen are bi-racial.

I, personally, consider, Dolly Parton, the sexiest woman alive. And how I would give anything, just, too "pardon" her.

To prove that you're mine, I will inscribe *my* "logo," on your behind.

It's a shame that, most, people *cannot* become uninhibited without the use of alcohol, or drugs.

More people derive "pleasure" from pain, than most people would want to believe.

Since people are rarely what they appear too be, never criticize anyone, to another, especially where one's sexuality is concerned.

Believe it or not, not everyone is *uncomfortable* with being in the "closet."

People lie to "themselves" about *who* they sleep with. What makes you think they're going to tell *you* the truth?

Today, if you play, you may not live long enough to pay. Think about it.

You do not have to "desire" one, "sexually," to engage in sex with them.

Making love in the back of a, flatbed-truck, while riding, at night, on the Interstate. Wow!

It's difficult for a heterosexual male to maintain a close friendship with a male that's gay; because- sooner or later- sex will become an issue, or, it will come into play.

Sex, and Lies, goes hand-in-hand. This is why I put very little credence in "sexual statistics."

I love it when she "yearns" for my sperm.

Would you believe that there are women that do not douche!

If you're doing it "right," then sex isn't something that you *need* every night.

What men consider "sexual-encounters," women consider "sexual relationships."

Make your own flag-poles: Take two sticks, and staple your clean, and pressed, underwear to one of them; and her clean, and pressed, panties too the other. You now have your own "his, and hers" personal flag-poles. Wave them with pride!

Don't buy a cologne that is popular, but one that is complementary to you.

There is sex and there is "sex-" oral- sex is the former, not the latter. Cause, if there isn't any penetration, there isn't <u>any</u> Indication.

Say it loud: I'm a "freak" and I'm proud!

My "love -tool is like the "starship enterprise:" It is, also, willing to go where *No Man* has gone before.

Share quiet moments together- just thinking, and listening, to your surrounding.

Be careful of what you give- sexually. For, what you give you will- sooner or later- want to receive. Think about it.

This is one of the biggest myths ever told: Telephone; Telegraph; Tell a "Woman." It should be: Telephone; Telegraph; Tell a "Man."

Let's not confuse one's "sexual experiences," with one's "sexual lifestyle."

It's a myth that a woman's vagina has no face. Because I have seen some pretty ugly ones in my time.

People are no longer just satisfied with what's going on in *your* bedroom. They want to know what's going on under *your* sheets as well.

A man should find nothing "kinder," than a "woman's vagina!

When you tell a woman that you "love her" she, automatically, interprets that to mean that you are "in-love" with her. The hardest thing for a man to do, is to tell a woman that he "loves her," but he's not, "in love," with her.

There is more "discrimination" between gays, themselves, than there is between heterosexuals and gays.

"If you *enjoyed* making them, then, you should, have no problem with taking care of them. "Who said that making them was, all, that enjoyable?"

While you're out there doing your thing on the "down-low," don't think that she's not back home doing the same.

Wine her, and Dine her, then bring her home, and "grind" her.

I love it when her eyes beam on my long, lean, "mean cuisine."

Be direct, and tell her what you want. After all, you can't get what you want, unless, you go after that which is wanted by you.

Sex- like politics and religion- is not only a *personal* issue, but a *profound* one as well. This is why it is too *complex* to be understood by anyone that's not of "legal age."

I've heard of Bi-curious. But, have you ever heard of: homo-curious, lesbi-curious, or hetero-curious?

How come heterosexuals seem to he curious about gays, lesbians and bisexuals? Yet, none of the above appear to be, *too,* curious about them.

Heterosexuals love their opposite sex; Gays and lesbians love their same sex; bisexuals, love both sexes. However, "freaks" just love "sex," and in *many* cases, anyone of age will do- even, though *most,* do have a "sexual preference."

What's worse than a woman pouting? An *oversized,* woman pouting.

Women will often use "bad relationships" with men as an *excuse* for them turning to other "women." However, men will rarely use "bad relationships," with women, as an *excuse* for them turning to other "men."

You have a *consenting* woman, and *three* consenting men- each of a *different* nationality. The woman wants all of them to make love to her at the same time. She will engage in oral-sex with one, vaginal-intercourse with, another, and anal intercourse with the other. Whoever wins the *toss* of the coin gets to plant *his* "flag-pole" wherever he desires, and when she is occupied by all- then, and only then, will the fun begin.

You're in an empty room, you're both naked, and you want to play a game. Well, here's a game: She plays the part of the matador-dangling a *"red cloth"* in front of you, and you are the "bull." Charge! Go get her "cowboy!" Need I say more?

Pretend that you are husband and wife; live together for a year; and do *all* the things that a married couple would, and *should,* do. Try this before you say: I do!

Women love bald headed men, because, they have *two* smooth "heads" to rub, rather than just one.

> *A*void
>   *I*n
>   *D*iscriminate
>   *S*ex

Say No, today, a*nd live* to say,Yes, tomorrow.

Sex is a thriller, and Aids is a killer. Protect yourself from this "trill-kill."

Soak her feet; dry her feet, and massage her feet. After all is done, go and apply whip cream to each one of her toes, and go, and suck, on each one of those "little- piggees." Hey! Go for yours.

I love it when she's on her knees, with her mouth opened wide, and just waiting for me to insert my "mean machine" into her mouth, so she can receive her, daily, shot of "liquid-love."

Why do many people feel the need to "publicly" announce their, sexuality. Why don't they just take care of business; keep *their* business to themselves; and, go on about *their* business.

To each, his own; provided it's kept in one's <u>own</u> home. What people don't know, they can't judge.

If God wanted "mankind" to <u>actively</u> <u>engage</u> in "bisexual behavior," He would have made each, and everyone of us, Hermaphrodite!

If you want Respect: Love <u>everyone</u>, but take "Crap" from <u>no</u> <u>one</u>. Then just sit back, and watch the women come!

If you criticize her with "pride," then you should, also, apologize to her with pride.

I'm not your "Ordinary;" but baby, I am <u>your</u> "Extraordinary."

When you drink you <u>can't</u> think. So think, and <u>don't</u> drink. Stay safe, healthy, and look out for each other.

Some men feel that they should cherish, and "worship" their woman. If you want to cherish her-fine. But don't worship her, or anyone else. Worship is reserved <u>only</u> for one's "Higher Power."

Dildos and vibrators may have their <u>place</u>, but make no mistake, cause, they cannot <u>replace</u>. Remember: There's nothing like the "real Thing," baby.

It's <u>your</u> Life; it's <u>your</u> Business; it's <u>your</u> Preference; it's <u>your</u> Body; and, it's <u>your</u> Memories. So, go for <u>yours</u>!

"I am neither gay, nor bisexual, but I did meet a girl once that was, so, attractive, I could have had a lesbian <u>experience</u> with her." This was told to me by a girl I once dated. Could she be considered: hetero-flexible?

When something goes wrong in an, intimate relationship, always blame the woman. Women were, after-all, created to take the blame for the "<u>inadequacies</u>" of men!

You did make a "mess" of things, but, now she's back in your bed, again; she claims she hears a symphony; and she's no longer saying : " she can't get no satisfaction." Mission accomplished!

With so many categories of "sexual references" out there, I guess it will be only a matter of time when heterosexuality will no longer be considered the "in thing," but rather, the "out thing." You know what they say: Nothing lasts forever!

It's quite evident that "we" are not all that, cause, if we were, women wouldn't be turning to women at such a rapid rate. We better open our eyes, and "smell the coffee."

In, most cases, two women engaging in a sexual act, with each other, is considered a "turn-on." Whereas, with, two, men it's considered a "turn-off." This proves that what is good for the goose, is not, always, good for the gander. Enough said for Equality.

Hepatitis, Herpes, and HIV: Trust me. You want to leave home without them.

Knowledge, and love *are* eternal – sex is not. Always keep this in mind.

Love yourself; Respect yourself; Protect yourself. This is your responsibility, so, don't you dare delegate it to somebody else.

"If your boy got a girl pregnant, what would you do?" Nothing! If he found a way in, I'm sure he can find a way out.

If someone, would, ask you: Are you gay, what would you say? I would tell them that on, Monday's and Tuesday's- I'm heterosexual; and on Wednesday's and Thursday's- I'm gay; and on Friday's and Saturday's- I'm bisexual; and on Sunday's- I'm asexual; cause, I need my rest, especially, from flip-flopping on Friday's and Saturday's.

Are you gay? Not today, but, maybe tomorrow! One never knows; and never say, never.

I prefer women of average height, and weight. However, I've been known to have women that were quite "hefty," and that was 'cool." It's like going to rent a car: You want to rent an average compact car, but the dealer only has "SUVs available. It beats the alternative (if you g rip where I'm coming from).

Your "home-boy" would bend over, and become your "honey," every-time he needed, some drug money. Are <u>you</u> willing to get "funny" for some money?

Buy condoms: They may set you back a few bucks, but, you are <u>definitely</u> worth it.

You're sleeping with Charlene and Ebony- yet, you told me, that I was "wonderful" in bed. Why did you lie? "Honey, you are "wonderful" in bed; and Charlene is "fantastic" in bed. But Ebony, well Ebony, she's "terrific" in bed. You see, honey, I did not lie to you. You <u>are</u> "wonderful" in bed."

After you bring her roses, make sure she, only, gets stuck by <u>your</u> "thorn."

Remember: A condom is a terrible thing to waste. Waste not, regret

What is a person that is <u>addicted</u> to Fellatio suffering from? "Prick-n-Mouth" disease!

Stand tall, take off all your clothes, and spread your legs, as wide as you can. Have your mate play the song "Limbo Rock" by Chubby Checker. Can she do the Limbo between your legs? Let's see. How low, do you think, she can go without touching the tip, of <u>your</u> "licorice-stick."

While your woman is breast-feeding your child with, one of her breasts, why don't you, at the same time, let <u>her</u> feed <u>you</u> with the other one. It's a "family affair," so, why munch elsewhere!

Let her slip on you the <u>flavored</u> condom of her choice, just before she performs oral-sex on you. After she gives it her best, she <u>will</u> confess, that it's the "sweetest thing" this side of heaven.

You're on a crowded bus; your lady is wearing a skirt that is zipped down in the rear; she's sitting on your lap; and your "erect wood" is inside of her throughout the entire ride. "Step up, and keep it moving, in the rear of the bus."

AIDS is <u>not</u> a curse from God. It's a curse from a group, of men, <u>trying</u> to play God.

We're riding on the "D" train to Harlem. And during the 59th, and 125th street express stop me, and my lady, engaged in the most "heated" sex, that we had ever engaged in, in the last car of that empty subway car: "All a board!"

Can't wait, then play it safe. Don't hesitate, just go on, and masturbate. "Oh, what a relief it is."

Sex <u>is</u> a part of life, and it should be enjoyed by <u>all</u>. If you are HIV positive, or have Herpes, you can, still, have an active, and enjoyable, sex-life. However, you <u>should</u> be cautious; you <u>must</u> protect yourself; and you <u>have</u> to practice, and engage in, safe-sex. Don't run from life, Live it!

She's kneeling before you; she takes your long-stem "mushroom" in her hand, and she starts to sing into it. What song is she singing? "I love to love you baby," by Donna Summer: "Who says the <u>truth</u> hurts!"

That virgin was harder to "crack" than the cellophane on a new CD.

Fruits: They can make sex not only *delicious*, but, also, quite *nutritious*, if one uses one's imagination.

Masturbate for your partner, from time to time, for this will help them to *further* understand your sexual desires.

Hey guys, ask your woman, from time to time: How *slick* is she willing to get, for your *stick*.

People, especially men, will do what they desire too do, and then attach a label, one that they can live with, to it. This is why we have terminology such as: Metro-sexual; Try-sexual; Hetero-flexible; Bi-curious, etc. Remember that a "rose," by any other name, is still a rose.

Perform *oral-sex,* on her, while she is standing on her head. Wow!

The only way anyone can make *you* doubt *your* sexuality, is if *you* doubt it *yourself.*

I don't know about you guys, but, I get turned on by *total* "firmness."

Cellulite is a *definite* turn-off.

I once dated a girl with a nose *so* long, and nostrils *so* wide, I, seriously, considered having "nostril Intercourse" with her. I'm a *freak*, so, sue me.

Guys, generally speaking- we are *more* "inhibited" than women.

I would love to spend a weekend, with my lady, in a *"nudist colony"*.

Please, do not wear *black* lipstick. Because it's a real turn-off.

I love women in "designer jeans." It's a *fit* made in "heaven."

I would *love* to make love on a flatbed train while it is moving on track.

I've always wondered: outside of sex do, *most,* men *genuinely* care for women.

Too many women today not only want their man to bring home the "bacon," but, they want him to cook it as well.

I'd love to take a pair of "Chinese chopsticks," and use them to play the drums on *her,* naked, buns. Her "buns" *will* come alive with the "sound of music."

If you're, bi-sexual, let me know. Do not assume that I probably wouldn't *want* you.

Once a woman *tries* to change me, it is quite evident that she wants someone *other* than me. Therefore, she has to go.

Using chewing gum, let's play "pin the tail" on the donkey. Your woman, of course, will *act* as the "donkey."

I love it when she tells me, that she can't believe that she ate *my* whole thing!

Believe it or not, guys do more "kissing and telling" than women. It's something that men should admit, and it's something that they should *STOP!*

I would love to perform on stage, and in the nude, during a "rock concert." What can I tell you: "I got that loving- feeling."

I want you to lie across my lap, on your stomach, and let me use your nude body, as a desk, to do my homework on.

If you think, *you're,* a "super freak," then read the works of, Marquis de Sade.

Once you hit a woman, you have, *voluntarily,* forfeited any respect as a "man."

I love it when she gives me a *"tongue bath"*

A woman that knows how to package herself is, in my opinion, quite desirable.

Whether you are the "top-man," or the "bottom-man," you are *both* active participants in the same act, and, <u>most</u> likely, will share "equal billing."

I knew someone who was gay, and had quite a few boyfriends. He decided to have a sex-change and proceeded with the process. To his dismay, he lost all of his boyfriends. They told him that if they had wanted to be with a female, they wouldn't have been with him. Why settle for a transsexual when you can have the "natural" thing.

What do you say to a Virgin when you're making-out, for the first time?
>Ooh, ooh love
>>I will pump, a <u>little,</u> easier
>Ooh, ooh love
>>You'll be a <u>little,</u> less, tighter

If your have any doubts, try this: you can be affectionate, and intimate, but, use a "sex toy," instead, to penetrate her, rather then your penis.

Stick <u>your</u> "key" in her lock, and don't stop turning until you've satisfied her "yearning."

They call me "Tiger," cause, I'm not <u>only</u> considered "great" in bed, but I, also, know how to swing <u>my</u> "Wood."

"I think you're bisexual. "I'll <u>Bi</u> that, but, then again, I'll <u>Bi</u> anything!

<u>Without exception</u>, God loves everyone!

"SEX IS WHAT A GOOD MEAL SHOULD BE"

MUSIC and LYRICS

Johnnie Newkirk Jr.

Special thanks to my music copyist, Steve Cohen.

SEX IS WHAT A GOOD MEAL SHOULD BE
Music and Lyrics By: Johnnie Newkirk Jr.

Chorus
Sex is what a good meal should be, that's delicious
and nutritious (repeat).

First, serve her an appetizer, before the main meal
After dessert, don't you forget to, serve her
something
that will, quench her thirst.

Chorus
Sex is what a good meal should be, that's delicious
and nutritious (repeat)

First, get to know her, before the first date.
When it's time, to slide into home base see, a
doctor and a minister, first
Hey, by the end of the day, listen to what I say.

Chorus
Sex is what a good meal should be, that's delicious
and nutritious (repeat)

Get to know each other
Respect one another
Protect yourself for each other
Stay true to one another

Sex Is What A Good Meal Should Be

**Music & Lyrics by
Johnnie Newkirk**

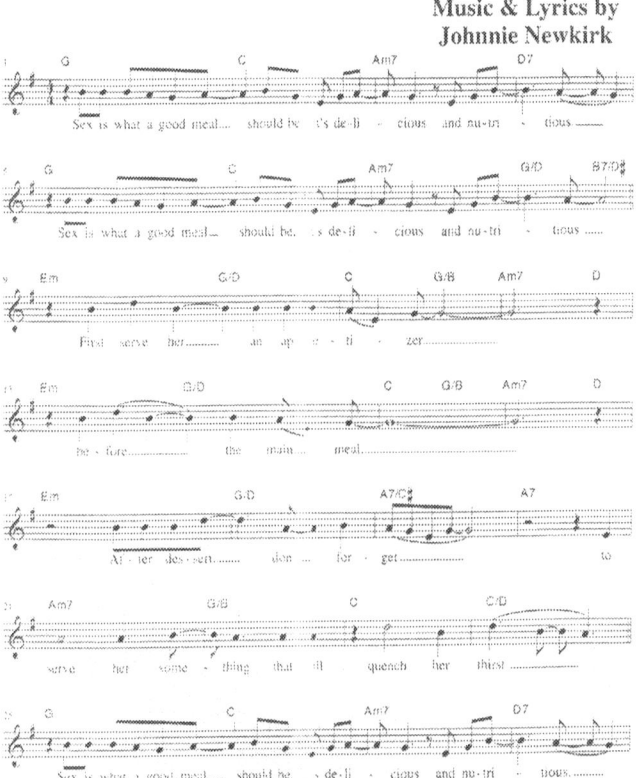

Johnnie Newkirk, Jr.

— 2 — Sex Is What A Good Meal Should Be

— 3 — Sex Is What A Good Meal Should Be

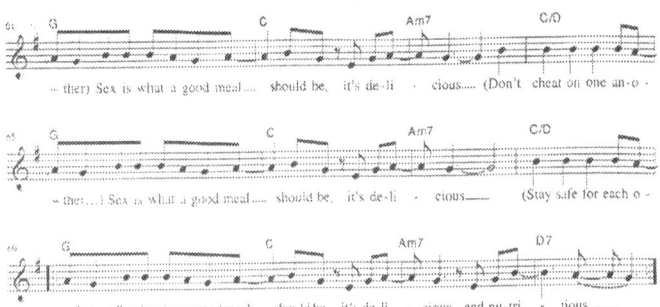

... ther) Sex is what a good meal.... should be, it's de-li · cious..... (Don't cheat on one an-o -

– ther...) Sex is what a good meal..... should be, it's de-li · cious....... (Stay safe for each o -

– ther...) Sex is what a good meal.... should be, it's de-li · cious and nu-tri · tious........

REPEAT & FADE

79

About the Author

Johnnie Newkirk, Jr. is a retired, certified, caseworker who has lived all his life in Brooklyn, New York. Johnnie is a fifty year-old widower who is currently single. He is a singer, composer, designer, and businessman who loves to read, write, walk, and watch old classics on television. He's founder/chairman of New West Music & Publishing.

www.NEWWESTMUSICPUBLISHING.com

We Are Making A Difference

You are important.

You do count.

You can be "You" with us.

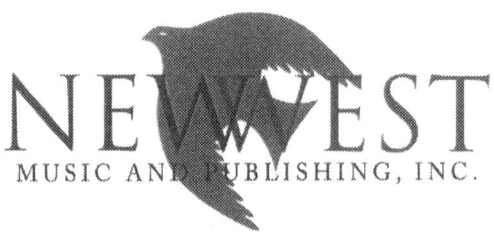

Recording Label
Publishing Company
Music Online
Books Online
Pamphlets Online
Free Posters Online
Free Articles Online
Sheet Music Online
Message Board
Faces of God